CH00690904

KETO DIET COOKBOOK

2021

MOUTH-WATERING RECIPES EASY TO MAKE FOR BEGINNERS

ADELE LECLERC

Table of Contents

Delicious Frittata

Try a keto frittata today! It's so tasty!

Preparation time: 10 minutes

Cooking time: 1 hour

Servings: 4

Ingredients:

- 9 ounces spinach
- 12 eggs
- 1-ounce pepperoni
- 1 teaspoon garlic, minced
- Salt and black pepper to the taste
- 5 ounces mozzarella, shredded
- ½ cup parmesan, grated
- ½ cup ricotta cheese
- 4 tablespoons olive oil
- A pinch of nutmeg

Directions:

1. Squeeze liquid from spinach and put in a bowl.

2. In another bowl, mix eggs with salt, pepper, nutmeg and garlic and whisk well.

3. Add spinach, parmesan and ricotta and whisk well again.

4. Pour this into a pan, sprinkle mozzarella and pepperoni on top, introduce in the oven and bake at 375 degrees F for 45 minutes.

5. Leave frittata to cool down for a few minutes before serving it.

Enjoy!

Nutrition: calories 298, fat 2, fiber 1, carbs 6, protein 18

Smoked Salmon Breakfast

It will surprise you with its taste!

Preparation time: 10 minutes

Cooking time: 10 minutes

Servings: 3

Ingredients:

- 4 eggs, whisked
- ½ teaspoon avocado oil
- 4 ounces smoked salmon, chopped
- *For the sauce:*
- 1 cup coconut milk
- ½ cup cashews, soaked, drained
- ¼ cup green onions, chopped
- 1 teaspoon garlic powder
- Salt and black pepper to the taste
- 1 tablespoon lemon juice

Directions:

1. In your blender, mix cashews with coconut milk, garlic powder and lemon juice and blend well.
2. Add salt, pepper and green onions, blend again well, transfer to a bowl and keep in the fridge for now.
3. Heat up a pan with the oil over medium-low heat, add eggs, whisk a bit and cook until they are almost done
4. Introduce in your preheated broiler and cook until eggs set.
5. Divide eggs on plates, top with smoked salmon and serve with the green onion sauce on top.

Enjoy!

Nutrition: calories 200, fat 10, fiber 2, carbs 11, protein 15

Feta And Asparagus Delight

These elements combine very well!

Preparation time: 10 minutes

Cooking time: 25 minutes

Servings: 2

Ingredients:

- 12 asparagus spears
- 1 tablespoon olive oil
- 2 green onions, chopped
- 1 garlic clove, minced
- 6 eggs
- Salt and black pepper to the taste
- ½ cup feta cheese

Directions:

1. Heat up a pan with some water over medium heat, add asparagus, cook for 8 minutes, drain well, chop 2 spears and reserve the rest.

2. Heat up a pan with the oil over medium heat, add garlic, chopped asparagus and onions, stir and cook for 5 minutes.
3. Add eggs, salt and pepper, stir, cover and cook for 5 minutes.
4. Arrange the whole asparagus on top of your frittata, sprinkle cheese, introduce in the oven at 350 degrees F and bake for 9 minutes.
5. Divide between plates and serve.

Enjoy!

Nutrition: calories 340, fat 12, fiber 3, carbs 8, protein 26

Special Breakfast Eggs

This is truly the best keto eggs recipe you can ever try!

Preparation time: 10 minutes

Cooking time: 4 minutes

Servings: 12

Ingredients:

- 4 tea bags
- 4 tablespoons salt
- 12 eggs
- 2 tablespoons cinnamon
- 6-star anise
- 1 teaspoon black pepper
- 1 tablespoons peppercorns
- 8 cups water
- 1 cup tamari sauce

Directions:

1. Put water in a pot, add eggs, bring them to a boil over medium heat and cook until they are hard boiled.
2. Cool them down and crack them without peeling.

3. In a large pot, mix water with tea bags, salt, pepper, peppercorns, cinnamon, star anise and tamari sauce.
4. Add cracked eggs, cover pot, bring to a simmer over low heat and cook for 30 minutes.
5. Discard tea bags and cook eggs for 3 hours and 30 minutes.
6. Leave eggs to cool down, peel and serve them for breakfast.

Enjoy!

Nutrition: calories 90, fat 6, fiber 0, carbs 0, protein 7

Eggs Baked In Avocados

They are so delicious and they look great too!

Preparation time: 10 minutes

Cooking time: 20 minutes

Servings: 4

Ingredients:

- 2 avocados, cut in halves and pitted
- 4 eggs
- Salt and black pepper to the taste
- 1 tablespoon chives, chopped

Directions:

1. Scoop some flesh from the avocado halves and arrange them in a baking dish.

2. Crack an egg in each avocado, season with salt and pepper, introduce them in the oven at 425 degrees F and bake for 20 minutes.
3. Sprinkle chives at the end and serve for breakfast!

Enjoy!

Nutrition: calories 400, fat 34, fiber 13, carbs 13, protein 15

Shrimp And Bacon Breakfast

This is a perfect breakfast idea!

Preparation time: 10 minutes

Cooking time: 15 minutes

Servings: 4

Ingredients:

- 1 cup mushrooms, sliced
- 4 bacon slices, chopped
- 4 ounces smoked salmon, chopped
- 4 ounces shrimp, deveined
- Salt and black pepper to the taste
- ½ cup coconut cream

Directions:

1. Heat up a pan over medium heat, add bacon, stir and cook for 5 minutes.
2. Add mushrooms, stir and cook for 5 minutes more.
3. Add salmon, stir and cook for 3 minutes.

4. Add shrimp and cook for 2 minutes.

5. Add salt, pepper and coconut cream, stir, cook for 1 minute, take off heat and divide between plates.

Enjoy!

Nutrition: calories 340, fat 23, fiber 1, carbs 4, protein 17

Delicious Mexican Breakfast

Try a Ketogenic Mexican breakfast today!

Preparation time: 10 minutes

Cooking time: 30 minutes

Servings: 8

Ingredients:

- ½ cup enchilada sauce
- 1 pound pork, ground
- 1 pound chorizo, chopped
- Salt and black pepper to the taste
- 8 eggs
- 1 tomato, chopped
- 3 tablespoons ghee
- ½ cup red onion, chopped
- 1 avocado, pitted, peeled and chopped

Directions:

1. In a bowl, mix pork with chorizo, stir and spread on a lined baking form.

2. Spread enchilada sauce on top, introduce in the oven at 350 degrees F and bake for 20 minutes.
3. Heat up a pan with the ghee over medium heat, add eggs and scramble them well.
4. Take pork mix out of the oven and spread scrambled eggs over them.
5. Sprinkle salt, pepper, tomato, onion and avocado, divide between plates and serve.

Enjoy!

Nutrition: calories 400, fat 32, fiber 4, carbs 7, protein 25

Delicious Breakfast Pie

Pay attention and learn how to make this great breakfast in no time!

Preparation time: 10 minutes

Cooking time: 45 minutes

Servings: 8

Ingredients:

- ½ onion, chopped
- 1 pie crust
- ½ red bell pepper, chopped
- ¾ pound beef, ground
- Salt and black pepper to the taste
- 3 tablespoons taco seasoning
- A handful cilantro, chopped
- 8 eggs
- 1 teaspoon coconut oil
- 1 teaspoon baking soda
- Mango salsa for serving

Directions:

1. Heat up a pan with the oil over medium heat, add beef, cook until it browns and mixes with salt, pepper and taco seasoning.
2. Stir again, transfer to a bowl and leave aside for now.
3. Heat up the pan again over medium heat with cooking juices from the meat, add onion and bell pepper, stir and cook for 4 minutes.
4. Add eggs, baking soda and some salt and stir well.
5. Add cilantro, stir again and take off heat.
6. Spread beef mix in pie crust, add veggies mix and spread over meat, introduce in the oven at 350 degrees F and bake for 45 minutes.
7. Leave the pie to cool down a bit, slice, divide between plates and serve with mango salsa on top.

Enjoy!

Nutrition: calories 198, fat 11, fiber 1, carbs 12, protein 12

Breakfast Stir Fry

We recommend you try this keto breakfast as soon as possible!

Preparation time: 10 minutes

Cooking time: 30 minutes

Servings: 2

Ingredients:

- ½ pounds beef meat, minced
- 2 teaspoons red chili flakes
- 1 tablespoon tamari sauce
- 2 bell peppers, chopped
- 1 teaspoon chili powder
- 1 tablespoon coconut oil
- Salt and black pepper to the taste

For the bok choy:

- 6 bunches bok choy, trimmed and chopped
- 1 teaspoon ginger, grated
- Salt to the taste
- 1 tablespoon coconut oil

For the eggs:

- 1 tablespoon coconut oil

- 2 eggs

Directions:

1. Heat up a pan with 1 tablespoon coconut oil over medium high heat, add beef and bell peppers, stir and cook for 10 minutes.
2. Add salt, pepper, tamari sauce, chili flakes and chili powder, stir, cook for 4 minutes more and take off heat.
3. Heat up another pan with 1 tablespoon oil over medium heat, add bok choy, stir and cook for 3 minutes.
4. Add salt and ginger, stir, cook for 2 minutes more and take off heat.
5. Heat up the third pan with 1 tablespoon oil over medium heat, crack eggs and fry them.
6. Divide beef and bell peppers mix into 2 bowls.
7. Divide bok choy and top with eggs.

Enjoy!

Nutrition: calories 248, fat 14, fiber 4, carbs 10, protein 14

Delicious Breakfast Skillet

It's going to be so tasty!

Preparation time: 10 minutes

Cooking time: 30 minutes

Servings: 4

Ingredients:

- 8 ounces mushrooms, chopped
- Salt and black pepper to the taste
- 1 pound pork, minced
- 1 tablespoon coconut oil
- ½ teaspoon garlic powder
- ½ teaspoon basil, dried
- 2 tablespoons Dijon mustard
- 2 zucchinis, chopped

Directions:

1. Heat up a pan with the oil over medium high heat, add mushrooms, stir and cook for 4 minutes.
2. Add zucchinis, salt and pepper, stir and cook for 4 minutes more.

3. Add pork, garlic powder, basil, more salt and pepper, stir and cook until meat is done.
4. Add mustard, stir, cook for 3 minutes more, divide into bowls and serve.

Enjoy!

Nutrition: calories 240, fat 15, fiber 2, carbs 9, protein 17

Breakfast Casserole

You've got to try this!

Preparation time: 10 minutes

Cooking time: 40 minutes

Servings: 4

Ingredients:

- 10 eggs
- 1 pound pork sausage, chopped
- 1 yellow onion, chopped
- 3 cups spinach, torn
- Salt and black pepper to the taste
- 3 tablespoons avocado oil

Directions:

1. Heat up a pan with 1 tablespoon oil over medium heat, add sausage, stir and brown it for 4 minutes.
2. Add onion, stir and cook for 3 minutes more.
3. Add spinach, stir and cook for 1 minute.
4. Grease a baking dish with the rest of the oil and spread sausage mix.

5. Whisk eggs and add them to sausage mix.

6. Stir gently, introduce in the oven at 350 degrees F and bake for 30 minutes.

7. Leave casserole to cool down for a few minutes before serving it for breakfast.

Enjoy!

Nutrition: calories 345, fat 12, fiber 1, carbs 8, protein 22

Incredible Breakfast Patties

This is incredibly tasty and easy to make for breakfast!

Preparation time: 10 minutes

Cooking time: 10 minutes

Servings: 4

Ingredients:

- 1 pound pork meat, minced
- Salt and black pepper to the taste
- ¼ teaspoon thyme, dried
- ½ teaspoon sage, dried
- ¼ teaspoon ginger, dried
- 3 tablespoon cold water
- 1 tablespoon coconut oil

Directions:

1. Put meat in a bowl.
2. In another bowl, mix water with salt, pepper, sage, thyme and ginger and whisk well.
3. Add this to meat and stir very well.
4. Shape your patties and place them on a working surface.

5. Heat up a pan with the coconut oil over medium high heat, add patties, fry them for 5 minutes, flip and cook them for 3 minutes more.
6. Serve them warm.

Enjoy!

Nutrition: calories 320, fat 13, fiber 2, carbs 10, protein 12

Delicious Sausage Quiche

It's so amazing! You must make it for breakfast tomorrow!

Preparation time: 10 minutes

Cooking time: 40 minutes

Servings: 6

Ingredients:

- 12 ounces pork sausage, chopped
- Salt and black pepper to the taste
- 2 teaspoons whipping cream
- 2 tablespoons parsley, chopped
- 10 mixed cherry tomatoes, halved
- 6 eggs
- 2 tablespoons parmesan, grated
- 5 eggplant slices

Directions:

1. Spread sausage pieces on the bottom of a baking dish.
2. Layer eggplant slices on top.
3. Add cherry tomatoes.

4. In a bowl, mix eggs with salt, pepper, cream and parmesan and whisk well.
5. Pour this into the baking dish, introduce in the oven at 375 degrees F and bake for 40 minutes.
6. Serve right away.

Enjoy!

Nutrition: calories 340, fat 28, fiber 3, carbs 3, protein 17

Special Breakfast Dish

This is a Ketogenic breakfast worth trying!

Preparation time: 10 minutes

Cooking time: 40 minutes

Servings: 6

Ingredients:

- 1 pound sausage, chopped
- 1 leek, chopped
- 8 eggs, whisked
- ¼ cup coconut milk
- 6 asparagus stalks, chopped
- 1 tablespoon dill, chopped
- Salt and black pepper to the taste
- ¼ teaspoon garlic powder
- 1 tablespoon coconut oil, melted

Directions:

1. Heat up a pan over medium heat, add sausage pieces and brown them for a few minutes.
2. Add asparagus and leek, stir and cook for a few minutes.

3. Meanwhile, in a bowl, mix eggs with salt, pepper, dill, garlic powder and coconut milk and whisk well.

4. Pour this into a baking dish which you've greased with the coconut oil.

5. Add sausage and veggies on top and whisk everything.

6. Introduce in the oven at 325 degrees F and bake for 40 minutes.

7. Serve warm.

Enjoy!

Nutrition: calories 340, fat 12, fiber 3, carbs 8, protein 23

Chorizo And Cauliflower Breakfast

You don't need to be an expert cook to make a great breakfast! Try this next recipe and enjoy!

Preparation time: 10 minutes

Cooking time: 45 minutes

Servings: 4

Ingredients:

- 1 pound chorizo, chopped
- 12 ounces canned green chilies, chopped
- 1 yellow onion, chopped
- ½ teaspoon garlic powder
- Salt and black pepper to the taste
- 1 cauliflower head, florets separated
- 4 eggs, whisked
- 2 tablespoons green onions, chopped

Directions:

1. Heat up a pan over medium heat, add chorizo and onion, stir and brown for a few minutes.

2. Add green chilies, stir, cook for a few minutes and take off heat.

3. In your food processor mix cauliflower with some salt and pepper and blend.

4. Transfer this to a bowl, add eggs, salt, pepper and garlic powder and whisk everything.

5. Add chorizo mix as well, whisk again and transfer everything to a greased baking dish.

6. Bake in the oven at 375 degrees F and bake for 40 minutes.

7. Leave casserole to cool down for a few minutes, sprinkle green onions on top, slice and serve.

Enjoy!

Nutrition: calories 350, fat 12, fiber 4, carbs 6, protein 20

Italian Spaghetti Casserole

Try an Italian Ketogenic breakfast today!

Preparation time: 10 minutes

Cooking time: 55 minutes

Servings: 4

Ingredients:

- 4 tablespoons ghee
- 1 squash, halved
- Salt and black pepper to the taste
- ½ cup tomatoes, chopped
- 2 garlic cloves, minced
- 1 cup yellow onion, chopped
- ½ teaspoon Italian seasoning
- 3 ounces Italian salami, chopped
- ½ cup kalamata olives, chopped
- 4 eggs
- A handful parsley, chopped

Directions:

1. Place squash halves on a lined baking sheet, season with salt and pepper, spread 1 tablespoon ghee over them, introduce in the oven at 400 degrees F and bake for 45 minutes.
2. Meanwhile, heat up a pan with the rest of the ghee over medium heat, add garlic, onions, salt and pepper, stir and cook for a couple of minutes.
3. Add salami and tomatoes, stir and cook for 10 minutes.
4. Add olives, stir and cook for a few minutes more.
5. Take squash halves out of the oven, scrape flesh with a fork and add over salami mix into the pan.
6. Stir, make 4 holes in the mix, crack an egg in each, season with salt and pepper, introduce pan in the oven at 400 degrees F and bake until eggs are done.
7. Sprinkle parsley on top and serve.

Enjoy!

Nutrition: calories 333, fat 23, fiber 4, carbs 12, protein 15

Simple Breakfast Porridge

This is just delicious!

Preparation time: 5 minutes

Cooking time: 10 minutes

Servings: 1

Ingredients:

- 1 teaspoon cinnamon powder
- A pinch of nutmeg
- ½ cup almonds, ground
- 1 teaspoon stevia
- ¾ cup coconut cream
- A pinch of cardamom, ground
- A pinch of cloves, ground

Directions:

1. Heat up a pan over medium heat, add coconut cream and heat up for a few minutes.
2. Add stevia and almonds and stir well for 5 minutes.

3. Add cloves, cardamom, nutmeg and cinnamon and stir well.

4. Transfer to a bowl and serve hot.

Enjoy!

Nutrition: calories 200, fat 12, fiber 4, carbs 8, protein 16

Delicious Granola

A Ketogenic breakfast granola is the best idea ever!

Preparation time: 10 minutes

Cooking time: 0 minutes

Servings: 2

Ingredients:

- 2 tablespoons chocolate, chopped
- 7 strawberries, chopped
- A splash of lemon juice
- 2 tablespoons pecans, chopped

Directions:

1. In a bowl, mix chocolate with strawberries, pecans and lemon juice.
2. Stir and serve cold.

Enjoy!

Nutrition: calories 200, fat 5, fiber 4, carbs 7, protein 8

Delicious Almond Cereal

It's a great way to start your day!

Preparation time: 5 minutes

Cooking time: 0 minutes.

Servings: 1

Ingredients:

- 2 tablespoons almonds, chopped
- 2 tablespoon pepitas, roasted
- 1/3 cup coconut milk
- 1 tablespoon chia seeds
- 1/3 cup water
- A handful blueberries
- 1 small banana, chopped

Directions:

1. In a bowl, mix chia seeds with coconut milk and leave aside for 5 minutes.
2. In your food processor, mix half of the pepitas with almonds and pulse them well.
3. Add this to chia seeds mix.

41

4. Also add the water and stir.

5. Top with the rest of the pepitas, banana pieces and blueberries and serve.

Enjoy!

Nutrition: calories 200, fat 3, fiber 2, carbs 5, protein 4

Great Breakfast Bowl

You will be surprised! It's amazing!

Preparation time: 5 minutes

Cooking time: 0 minutes

Servings: 1

Ingredients:

- 1 teaspoon pecans, chopped
- 1 cup coconut milk
- 1 teaspoon walnuts, chopped
- 1 teaspoon pistachios, chopped
- 1 teaspoon almonds, chopped
- 1 teaspoon pine nuts, raw
- 1 teaspoon sunflower seeds, raw
- 1 teaspoon raw honey
- 1 teaspoon pepitas, raw
- 2 teaspoons raspberries

Directions:

1. In a bowl, mix milk with honey and stir.
2. Add pecans, walnuts, almonds, pistachios, sunflower seeds, pine nuts and pepitas.
3. Stir, top with raspberries and serve.

Enjoy!

Nutrition: calories 100, fat 2, fiber 4, carbs 5, protein 6

Delightful Breakfast Bread

This is a Ketogenic breakfast idea you should try soon!

Preparation time: 10 minutes

Cooking time: 3 minutes

Servings: 4

Ingredients:

- ½ teaspoon baking powder
- 1/3 cup almond flour
- 1 egg, whisked
- A pinch of salt
- 2 and ½ tablespoons coconut oil

Directions:

1. Grease a mug with some of the oil.
2. In a bowl, mix the egg with flour, salt, oil and baking powder and stir.
3. Pour this into the mug and cook in your microwave for 3 minutes at a High temperature.

4. Leave the bread to cool down a bit, take out of the mug, slice and serve with a glass of almond milk for breakfast.

Enjoy!

Nutrition: calories 132, fat 12, fiber 1, carbs 3, protein 4

Breakfast Muffins

These will really make your day much easier!

Preparation time: 10 minutes

Cooking time: 30 minutes

Servings: 4

Ingredients:

- ½ cup almond milk
- 6 eggs
- 1 tablespoon coconut oil
- Salt and black pepper to the taste
- ¼ cup kale, chopped
- 8 prosciutto slices
- ¼ cup chives, chopped

Directions:

1. In a bowl, mix eggs with salt, pepper, milk, chives and kale and stir well.
2. Grease a muffin tray with melted coconut oil, line with prosciutto slices, pour eggs mix, introduce in the oven and bake at 350 degrees F for 30 minutes.

3. Transfer muffins to a platter and serve for breakfast. Enjoy!

Nutrition: calories 140, fat 3, fiber 1, carbs 3, protein 10

Special Breakfast Bread

It's a Ketogenic breakfast bread full of nutrients!

Preparation time: 10 minutes

Cooking time: 25 minutes

Servings: 7

Ingredients:

- 1 cauliflower head, florets separated
- A handful parsley, chopped
- 1 cup spinach, torn
- 1 small yellow onion, chopped
- 1 tablespoon coconut oil
- ½ cup pecans, ground
- 3 eggs
- 2 garlic cloves, minced
- Salt and black pepper to the taste

Directions:

1. In your food processor, mix cauliflower florets with some salt and pepper and pulse well.
2. Heat up a pan with the oil over medium heat, add cauliflower, onion, garlic some salt and pepper, stir and cook for 10 minutes.
3. In a bowl, mix eggs with salt, pepper, parsley, spinach and nuts and stir.
4. Add cauliflower mix and stir well again.
5. Spread this into 7 rounds on a baking sheet, heat up the oven to 350 degrees F and bake for 15 minutes.
6. Serve these tasty breads for breakfast.

Enjoy!

Nutrition: calories 140, fat 3, fiber 3, carbs 4, protein 8

Breakfast Sandwich

It's a tasty Ketogenic breakfast sandwich! Try it soon!

Preparation time: 10 minutes

Cooking time: 10 minutes

Servings: 1

Ingredients:

- 2 eggs
- Salt and black pepper to the taste
- 2 tablespoons ghee
- ¼ pound pork sausage meat, minced
- ¼ cup water
- 1 tablespoon guacamole

Directions:

1. In a bowl, mix minced sausage meat with salt and pepper to the taste and stir well.
2. Shape a patty from this mix and place on a working surface.

3. Heat up a pan with 1 tablespoon ghee over medium heat, add sausage patty, fry for 3 minutes on each side and transfer to a plate.
4. Crack an egg in 2 bowls and whisk them a bit with some salt and pepper.
5. Heat up a pan with the rest of the ghee over medium high heat, place 2 biscuit cutters which you've greased with some ghee before in the pan and pour an egg in each.
6. Add the water to the pan, reduce heat, cover pan and cook eggs for 3 minutes.
7. Transfer these egg "buns" to paper towels and drain grease.
8. Place sausage patty on one egg "bun" spread guacamole over it and top with the other egg "bun".

Enjoy!

Nutrition: calories 200, fat 4, fiber 6, carbs 5, protein 10

Delicious Chicken Breakfast Muffins

It's a savory Ketogenic breakfast you can try today!

Preparation time: 10 minutes

Cooking time: 1 hour

Servings: 3

Ingredients:

- ¾ pound chicken breast, boneless
- Salt and black pepper to the taste
- ½ teaspoon garlic powder
- 3 tablespoons hot sauce mixed with 3 tablespoons melted coconut oil
- 6 eggs
- 2 tablespoons green onions, chopped

Directions:

1. Season chicken breast with salt, pepper and garlic powder, place on a lined baking sheet and bake in the oven at 425 degrees F for 25 minutes.
2. Transfer chicken breast to a bowl, shred with a fork and mix with half of the hot sauce and melted coconut oil.

3. Toss to coat and leave aside for now.

4. In a bowl, mix eggs with salt, pepper, green onions and the rest of the hot sauce mixed with oil and whisk very well.

5. Divide this mix into a muffin tray, top each with shredded chicken, introduce in the oven at 350 degrees F and bake for 30 minutes.

6. Serve your muffins hot.

Enjoy!

Nutrition: calories 140, fat 8, fiber 1, carbs 2, protein 13

Delicious Herbed Biscuits

Try this healthy keto breakfast biscuits really soon! They are so delicious!

Preparation time: 10 minutes

Cooking time: 15 minutes

Servings: 6

Ingredients:

- 6 tablespoons coconut oil
- 6 tablespoons coconut flour
- 2 garlic cloves, minced
- ¼ cup yellow onion, minced
- 2 eggs
- Salt and black pepper to the taste
- 1 tablespoons parsley, chopped
- 2 tablespoons coconut milk
- ½ teaspoon apple cider vinegar
- ¼ teaspoon baking soda

Directions:

1. In a bowl, mix coconut flour with eggs, oil, garlic, onion, coconut milk, parsley, salt and pepper and stir well.
2. In a bowl, mix vinegar with baking soda, stir well and add to the batter.
3. Drop spoonful of this batter on lined baking sheets and shape circles.
4. Introduce in the oven at 350 degrees F and bake for 15 minutes.
5. Serve these biscuits for breakfast.

Enjoy!

Nutrition: calories 140, fat 6, fiber 2, carbs 10, protein 12

Avocado Muffins

If you like avocado recipes, then you should really try this next one soon!

Preparation time: 10 minutes

Cooking time: 20 minutes

Servings: 12

Ingredients:

- 4 eggs
- 6 bacon slices, chopped
- 1 yellow onion, chopped
- 1 cup coconut milk
- 2 cups avocado, pitted, peeled and chopped
- Salt and black pepper to the taste
- ½ teaspoon baking soda
- ½ cup coconut flour

Directions:

1. Heat up a pan over medium heat, add onion and bacon, stir and brown for a few minutes.

2. In a bowl, mash avocado pieces with a fork and whisk well with the eggs.
3. Add milk, salt, pepper, baking soda and coconut flour and stir everything.
4. Add bacon mix and stir again.
5. Grease a muffin tray with the coconut oil, divide eggs and avocado mix into the tray, introduce in the oven at 350 degrees F and bake for 20 minutes.
6. Divide muffins between plates and serve them for breakfast.

Enjoy!

Nutrition: calories 200, fat 7, fiber 4, carbs 7, protein 5

Bacon And Lemon Breakfast Muffins

We are sure you've never tried something like this before! It's a

perfect keto breakfast!

Preparation time: 10 minutes

Cooking time: 20 minutes

Servings: 12

Ingredients:

- 1 cup bacon, finely chopped
- Salt and black pepper to the taste
- ½ cup ghee, melted
- 3 cups almond flour
- 1 teaspoon baking soda
- 4 eggs
- 2 teaspoons lemon thyme

Directions:

1. In a bowl, mix flour with baking soda and eggs and stir well.
2. Add ghee, lemon thyme, bacon, salt and pepper and whisk well.
3. Divide this into a lined muffin pan, introduce in the oven at 350 degrees F and bake for 20 minutes.
4. Leave muffins to cool down a bit, divide between plates and serve them.

Enjoy!

Nutrition: calories 213, fat 7, fiber 2, carbs 9, protein 8

Cheese And Oregano Muffins

We will make you love keto muffins from now on!

Preparation time: 10 minutes

Cooking time: 25 minutes

Servings: 6

Ingredients:

- 2 tablespoons olive oil
- 1 egg
- 2 tablespoons parmesan cheese
- ½ teaspoon oregano, dried
- 1 cup almond flour
- ¼ teaspoon baking soda
- Salt and black pepper to the taste
- ½ cup coconut milk
- 1 cup cheddar cheese, grated

Directions:

1. In a bowl, mix flour with oregano, salt, pepper, parmesan and baking soda and stir.
2. In another bowl, mix coconut milk with egg and olive oil and stir well.
3. Combine the 2 mixtures and whisk well.
4. Add cheddar cheese, stir, pour this a lined muffin tray, introduce in the oven at 350 degrees F for 25 minutes.
5. Leave your muffins to cool down for a few minutes, divide them between plates and serve.

Enjoy!

Nutrition: calories 160, fat 3, fiber 2, carbs 6, protein 10

Lunch Stuffed Peppers

These are perfect for a Ketogenic lunch!

Preparation time: 10 minutes

Cooking time: 40 minutes

Servings: 4

Ingredients:

- 4 big banana peppers, tops cut off, seeds removed and cut into halves lengthwise
- 1 tablespoon ghee
- Salt and black pepper to the taste
- ½ teaspoon herbs de Provence
- 1 pound sweet sausage, chopped
- 3 tablespoons yellow onions, chopped
- Some marinara sauce
- A drizzle of olive oil

Directions:

1. Season banana peppers with salt and pepper, drizzle the oil, rub well and bake in the oven at 350 degrees F for 20 minutes.

2. Meanwhile, heat up a pan over medium heat, add sausage pieces, stir and cook for 5 minutes.

3. Add onion, herbs de Provence, salt, pepper and ghee, stir well and cook for 5 minutes.

4. Take peppers out of the oven, fill them with the sausage mix, place them in an oven-proof dish, drizzle marinara sauce over them, introduce in the oven again and bake for 10 minutes more.

5. Serve hot.

Enjoy!

Nutrition: calories 320, fat 8, fiber 4, carbs 3, protein 10

Special Lunch Burgers

These burgers are really something very special!

Preparation time: 10 minutes

Cooking time: 25 minutes

Servings: 8

Ingredients:

- 1 pound brisket, ground
- 1 pound beef, ground
- Salt and black pepper to the taste
- 8 butter slices
- 1 tablespoon garlic, minced
- 1 tablespoon Italian seasoning
- 2 tablespoons mayonnaise
- 1 tablespoon ghee
- 2 tablespoons olive oil
- 1 yellow onion, chopped
- 1 tablespoon water

Directions:

1. In a bowl, mix brisket with beef, salt, pepper, Italian seasoning, garlic and mayo and stir well.
2. Shape 8 patties and make a pocket in each.
3. Stuff each burger with a butter slice and seal.
4. Heat up a pan with the olive oil over medium heat, add onions, stir and cook for 2 minutes.
5. Add the water, stir and gather them in the corner of the pan.
6. Place burgers in the pan with the onions and cook them over medium-low heat for 10 minutes.
7. Flip them, add the ghee and cook them for 10 minutes more.
8. Divide burgers on buns and serve them with caramelized onions on top.

Enjoy!

Nutrition: calories 180, fat 8, fiber 1, carbs 4, protein 20

Different Burger

serve this burger with the sauce we recommend you and enjoy!

Preparation time: 10 minutes

Cooking time: 30 minutes

Servings: 4

Ingredients:

For the sauce:

- 4 chili peppers, chopped
- 1 cup water
- 1 cup almond butter
- 1 teaspoon swerve
- 6 tablespoons coconut aminos
- 4 garlic cloves, minced
- 1 tablespoon rice vinegar

For the burgers:

- 4 pepper jack cheese slices
- 1 and ½ pounds beef, ground
- 1 red onion, sliced
- 8 bacon slices
- 8 lettuce leaves

- Salt and black pepper to the taste

Directions:

1. Heat up a pan with the almond butter over medium heat.
2. Add water, stir well and bring to a simmer.
3. Add coconut aminos and stir well.
4. In your food processor, mix chili peppers with garlic, swerve and vinegar and blend well.
5. Add this to almond butter mix, stir well, take off heat and leave aside for now.
6. In a bowl, mix beef with salt and pepper, stir and shape 4 patties.
7. Place them in a pan, introduce in your preheated broiler and broil for 7 minutes.
8. Flip burgers and broil them for 7 minutes more.
9. Place cheese slices on burgers, introduce in your broiler and broil for 4 minutes more.
10. Heat up a pan over medium heat, add bacon slices and fry them for a couple of minutes.

11.Place 2 lettuce leaves on a dish, add 1 burger on top, then 1 onion slice and 1 bacon slice and top with some almond butter sauce.

12.Repeat with the rest of the lettuce leaves, burgers, onion, bacon and sauce.

Enjoy!

Nutrition: calories 700, fat 56, fiber 10, carbs 7, protein 40

Delicious Zucchini Dish

It's easy to make and very light! Try this lunch dish soon!

Preparation time: 10 minutes

Cooking time: 5 minutes

Servings: 1

Ingredients:

- 1 tablespoon olive oil
- 3 tablespoons ghee
- 2 cups zucchini, cut with a spiralizer
- 1 teaspoon red pepper flakes
- 1 tablespoon garlic, minced
- 1 tablespoon red bell pepper, chopped
- Salt and black pepper to the taste
- 1 tablespoon basil, chopped
- ¼ cup asiago cheese, shaved
- ¼ cup parmesan, grated

Directions:

1. Heat up a pan with the oil and ghee over medium heat, add garlic, bell pepper and pepper flakes, stir and cook for 1 minute.
2. Add zucchini noodles, stir and cook for 2 minutes more.
3. Add basil, parmesan, salt and pepper, stir and cook for a few seconds more.
4. Take off heat, transfer to a bowl and serve for lunch with asiago cheese on top.

Enjoy!

Nutrition: calories 140, fat 3, fiber 1, carbs 1.3, protein 5

Bacon And Zucchini Noodles Salad

It's so refreshing and healthy! We adore this salad!

Preparation time: 10 minutes

Cooking time: 0 minutes

Servings: 2

Ingredients:

- 1 cup baby spinach
- 4 cups zucchini noodles
- 1/3 cup bleu cheese, crumbled
- 1/3 cup thick cheese dressing
- ½ cup bacon, cooked and crumbled
- Black pepper to the taste

Directions:

1. In a salad bowl, mix spinach with zucchini noodles, bacon and bleu cheese and toss.
2. Add cheese dressing and black pepper to the taste, toss well to coat, divide into 2 bowls and serve.

Enjoy!

Nutrition: calories 200, fat 14, fiber 4, carbs 2, protein 10

Amazing Chicken Salad

The best chicken salad you could taste is now available for you!

Preparation time: 10 minutes

Cooking time: 0 minutes

Servings: 3

Ingredients:

- 1 green onion, chopped
- 1 celery rib, chopped
- 1 egg, hard-boiled, peeled and chopped
- 5 ounces chicken breast, roasted and chopped
- 2 tablespoons parsley, chopped
- ½ tablespoons dill relish
- Salt and black pepper to the taste
- 1/3 cup mayonnaise
- A pinch of granulated garlic
- 1 teaspoon mustard

Directions:

1. In your food processor, mix parsley with onion and celery and pulse well.
2. Transfer these to a bowl and leave aside for now.
3. Put chicken meat in your food processor, blend well and add to the bowl with the veggies.
4. Add egg pieces, salt and pepper and stir.
5. Also add mustard, mayo, dill relish and granulated garlic, toss to coat and serve right away.

Enjoy!

Nutrition: calories 283, fat 23, fiber 5, carbs 3, protein 12

Unbelievable Steak Salad

If you are not in the mood for a Ketogenic chicken salad, then try a steak one instead!

Preparation time: 10 minutes

Cooking time: 20 minutes

Servings: 4

Ingredients:

- 1 and ½ pound steak, thinly sliced
- 3 tablespoons avocado oil
- Salt and black pepper to the taste
- ¼ cup balsamic vinegar
- 6 ounces sweet onion, chopped
- 1 lettuce head, chopped
- 2 garlic cloves, minced
- 4 ounces mushrooms, sliced
- 1 avocado, pitted, peeled and sliced
- 3 ounces sun-dried tomatoes, chopped
- 1 yellow bell pepper, sliced
- 1 orange bell pepper, sliced

- 1 teaspoon Italian seasoning
- 1 teaspoon red pepper flakes
- 1 teaspoon onion powder

Directions:

1. In a bowl, mix steak pieces with some salt, pepper and balsamic vinegar, toss to coat and leave aside for now.
2. Heat up a pan with the avocado oil over medium-low heat, add mushrooms, garlic, salt, pepper and onion, stir and cook for 20 minutes.
3. In a bowl, mix lettuce leaves with orange and yellow bell pepper, sun dried tomatoes and avocado and stirred.
4. Season steak pieces with onion powder, pepper flakes and Italian seasoning.
5. Place steak pieces in a broiling pan, introduce in preheated broiler and cook for 5 minutes.
6. Divide steak pieces on plates, add lettuce and avocado salad on the side and top everything with onion and mushroom mix.

Enjoy!

Nutrition: calories 435, fat 23, fiber 7, carbs 10, protein 35

Fennel and Chicken Lunch Salad

Try each day a different lunch salad! Today, we suggest you try this fennel and chicken delight!

Preparation time: 10 minutes

Cooking time: 0 minutes

Servings: 4

Ingredients:

- 3 chicken breasts, boneless, skinless, cooked and chopped
- 2 tablespoons walnut oil
- ¼ cup walnuts, toasted and chopped
- 1 and ½ cup fennel, chopped
- 2 tablespoons lemon juice
- ¼ cup mayonnaise
- 2 tablespoons fennel fronds, chopped
- Salt and black pepper to the taste
- A pinch of cayenne pepper

Directions:

1. In a bowl, mix fennel with chicken and walnuts and stir.
2. In another bowl, mix mayo with salt, pepper, fennel fronds, walnut oil, lemon juice, cayenne and garlic and stir well.
3. Pour this over chicken and fennel mix, toss to coat well and keep in the fridge until you serve.

Enjoy!

Nutrition: calories 200, fat 10, fiber 1, carbs 3, protein 7

Easy Stuffed Avocado

it's so easy to make for lunch!

Preparation time: 10 minutes

Cooking time: 0 minutes

Servings: 1

Ingredients:

- 1 avocado
- 4 ounces canned sardines, drained
- 1 spring onion, chopped
- 1 tablespoon mayonnaise
- 1 tablespoon lemon juice
- Salt and black pepper to the taste
- ¼ teaspoon turmeric powder

Directions:

1. Cut avocado in halves, scoop flesh and put in a bowl.

2. Mash with a fork and mix with sardines.

3. Mash again with your fork and mix with onion, lemon juice, turmeric powder, salt, pepper and mayo.

4. Stir everything and divide into avocado halves.

5. Serve for lunch right away.

Enjoy!

Nutrition: calories 230, fat 34, fiber 12, carbs 5, protein 27

Pesto Chicken Salad

The combination is absolutely delicious! You should try it!

Preparation time: 10 minutes

Cooking time: 0 minutes

Servings: 4

Ingredients:

- 1 pound chicken meat, cooked and cubed
- Salt and black pepper to the taste
- 10 cherry tomatoes, halved
- 6 bacon slices, cooked and crumbled
- ¼ cup mayonnaise
- 1 avocado, pitted, peeled and cubed
- 2 tablespoons garlic pesto

Directions:

1. In a salad bowl, mix chicken with bacon, avocado, tomatoes, salt and pepper and stir.
2. Add mayo and garlic pesto, toss well to coat and serve.

Enjoy!

Nutrition: calories 357, fat 23, fiber 5, carbs 3, protein 26

Tasty Lunch Salad

It's delicious and you will adore it once you try it!

Preparation time: 10 minutes

Cooking time: 10 minutes

Servings: 1

Ingredients:

- 4 ounces beef steak
- 2 cups lettuce leaves, shredded
- Salt and black pepper to the taste
- Cooking spray
- 2 tablespoons cilantro, chopped
- 2 radishes, sliced
- 1/3 cup red cabbage, shredded
- 3 tablespoons jarred chimichurri sauce
- 1 tablespoons salad dressing

For the salad dressing:

- 3 garlic cloves, minced
- ½ teaspoon Worcestershire sauce
- 1 tablespoon mustard
- ½ cup apple cider vinegar
- ¼ cup water

- ½ cup olive oil
- ¼ teaspoon Tabasco sauce
- Salt and black pepper to the taste

Directions:

1. In a bowl, mix garlic cloves with Worcestershire sauce, mustard, cider vinegar, water, olive oil, salt, pepper and Tabasco sauce, whisk well and leave aside for now.
2. Heat up your kitchen grill over medium high heat, spray cooking oil, add steak, season with salt and pepper, cook for 4 minutes, flip, cook for 4 minutes more, take off heat, leave aside to cool down and cut into thin strips.
3. In a salad bowl, mix lettuce with cilantro, cabbage, radishes, chimichurri sauce and steak strips.
4. Add 1 tablespoons of salad dressing, toss to coat and serve right away.

Enjoy!

Nutrition: calories 456, fat 32, fiber 2, carbs 6, protein 30

Easy Lunch Crab Cakes

Try these crab cakes for lunch! You won't regret it!

Preparation time: 10 minutes

Cooking time: 12 minutes

Servings: 6

Ingredients:

- 1 pound crabmeat
- ¼ cup parsley, chopped
- Salt and black pepper to the taste
- 2 green onions, chopped
- ¼ cup cilantro, chopped
- 1 teaspoon jalapeno pepper, minced
- 1 teaspoon lemon juice
- 1 teaspoon Worcestershire sauce
- 1 teaspoon old bay seasoning
- ½ teaspoon mustard powder
- ½ cup mayonnaise
- 1 egg
- 2 tablespoons olive oil

Directions:

1. In a large bowl mix crab meat with salt, pepper, parsley, green onions, cilantro, jalapeno, lemon juice, old bay seasoning, mustard powder and Worcestershire sauce and stir very well.
2. In another bowl mix egg wit mayo and whisk.
3. Add this to crabmeat mix and stir everything.
4. Shape 6 patties from this mix and place them on a plate.
5. Heat up a pan with the oil over medium high heat, add 3 crab cakes, cook for 3 minutes, flip, cook them for 3 minutes more and transfer to paper towels.
6. Repeat with the other 3 crab cakes, drain excess grease and serve for lunch.

Enjoy!

Nutrition: calories 254, fat 17, fiber 1, carbs 1, protein 20

Easy Lunch Muffins

These muffins will really get to your soul!

Preparation time: 10 minutes

Cooking time: 45 minutes

Servings: 13

Ingredients:

- 6 egg yolks
- 2 tablespoons coconut aminos
- ½ pound mushrooms
- ¾ cup coconut flour
- 1 pound beef, ground
- Salt to the taste

Directions:

1. In your food processor, mix mushrooms with salt, coconut aminos and egg yolks and blend well.
2. In a bowl, mix beef meat with some salt and stir.
3. Add mushroom mix to beef and stir everything.
4. Add coconut flour and stir again.

5. Divide this into 13 cupcake cups, introduce in the oven at 350 degrees f and bake for 45 minutes.

6. Serve them for lunch!

Enjoy!

Nutrition: calories 160, fat 10, fiber 3, carbs 1, protein 12

Lunch Pork Pie

This is something you've been craving for a very long time! Don't worry! It's a keto idea!

Preparation time: 10 minutes

Cooking time: 50 minutes

Servings: 6

Ingredients:

For the pie crust:

- 2 cups cracklings
- ¼ cup flax meal
- 1 cup almond flour
- 2 eggs
- A pinch of salt

For the filling:

- 1 cup cheddar cheese, grated
- 4 eggs
- 12 ounces pork loin, chopped
- 6 bacon slices
- ½ cup cream cheese
- 1 red onion, chopped

- ¼ cup chives, chopped
- 2 garlic cloves, minced
- Salt and black pepper to the taste
- 2 tablespoons ghee

Directions:

1. In your food processor, mix cracklings with almond flour, flax meal, 2 eggs and salt and blend until you obtain a dough.
2. Transfer this to a pie pan and press well on the bottom.
3. Introduce in the oven at 350 degrees F and bake for 15 minutes.
4. Meanwhile, heat up a pan with the ghee over medium high heat, add garlic and onion, stir and cook for 5 minutes.
5. Add bacon, stir and cook for 5 minutes.
6. Add pork loin, cook until it's brown on all sides and take off heat.
7. In a bowl, mix eggs with salt, pepper, cheddar cheese and cream cheese and blend well.

8. Add chives and stir again.

9. Spread pork into pie pan, add eggs mix, introduce in the oven at 350 degrees F and bake for 25 minutes.

10. Leave the pie to cool down for a couple of minutes and serve.

Enjoy!

Nutrition: calories 455, fat 34, fiber 3, carbs 3, protein 33

Delicious Lunch Pate

Enjoy something really easy to launch: a Ketogenic liver pate!

Preparation time: 10 minutes

Cooking time: 0 minutes

Servings: 1

Ingredients:

- 4 ounces chicken livers, sautéed
- 1 teaspoon mixed thyme, sage and oregano, chopped
- Salt and black pepper to the taste
- 3 tablespoons butter
- 3 radishes, thinly sliced
- Crusted bread slices for serving

Directions:

1. In your food processor, mix chicken livers with thyme, sage, oregano, butter, salt and pepper and blend very well for a few minutes.
2. Spread on crusted bread slices and top with radishes slices.
3. Serve right away.

Enjoy!

Nutrition: calories 380, fat 40, fiber 5, carbs 1, protein 17

Delicious Lunch Chowder

You might end up adoring this chowder! Try it at least once!

Preparation time: 10 minutes

Cooking time: 4 hours

Servings: 4

Ingredients:

- 1 pound chicken thighs, skinless and boneless
- 10 ounces canned tomatoes, chopped
- 1 cup chicken stock
- 8 ounces cream cheese
- Juice from 1 lime
- Salt and black pepper to the taste
- 1 jalapeno pepper, chopped
- 1 yellow onion, chopped
- 2 tablespoons cilantro, chopped
- 1 garlic clove, minced
- Cheddar cheese, shredded for serving
- Lime wedges for serving

Directions:

1. In your crock pot, mix chicken with tomatoes, stock, cream cheese, salt, pepper, lime juice, jalapeno, onion, garlic and cilantro, stir, cover and cook on High for 4 hours.

2. Uncover pot, shred meat into the pot, divide into bowls and serve with cheddar cheese on top and lime wedges on the side.

Enjoy!

Nutrition: calories 300, fat 5, fiber 6, carbs 3, protein 26

Delicious Coconut Soup

Try this Ketogenic coconut soup really soon! Everyone will love it!

Preparation time: 10 minutes

Cooking time: 30 minutes

Servings: 2

Ingredients:

- 4 cups chicken stock
- 3 lime leaves
- 1 and ½ cups coconut milk
- 1 teaspoon lemongrass, dried
- 1 cup cilantro, chopped
- 1 inch ginger, grated
- 4 Thai chilies, dried and chopped
- Salt and black pepper to the taste
- 4 ounces shrimp, raw, peeled and deveined
- 2 tablespoons red onion, chopped
- 1 tablespoon coconut oil
- 2 tablespoons mushrooms, chopped
- 1 tablespoon fish sauce

- 1 tablespoon cilantro, chopped
- Juice from 1 lime

Directions:

1. In a pot, mix chicken stock with coconut milk, lime leaves, lemongrass, Thai chilies, 1 cup cilantro, ginger, salt and pepper, stir, bring to a simmer over medium heat, cook for 20 minutes, strain and return to pot.
2. Heat up soup again over medium heat, add coconut oil, shrimp, fish sauce, mushrooms and onions, stir and cook for 10 minutes more.
3. Add lime juice and 1 tablespoon cilantro, stir, ladle into bowls and serve for lunch!

Enjoy!

Nutrition: calories 450, fat 34, fiber 4, carbs 8, protein 12

Zucchini Noodles Soup

This Ketogenic soup is simple and very tasty!

Preparation time: 10 minutes

Cooking time: 15 minutes

Servings: 8

Ingredients:

- 1 small yellow onion, chopped
- 2 garlic cloves, minced
- 1 jalapeno pepper, chopped
- 1 tablespoon coconut oil
- 1 and ½ tablespoons curry paste
- 6 cups chicken stock
- 15 ounces canned coconut milk
- 1 pound chicken breasts, sliced
- 1 red bell pepper, sliced
- 2 tablespoons fish sauce
- 2 zucchinis, cut with a spiralizer
- ½ cup cilantro, chopped
- Lime wedges for serving

Directions:

1. Heat up a pot with the oil over medium heat, add onion, stir and cook for 5 minutes.
2. Add garlic, jalapeno and curry paste, stir and cook for 1 minute.
3. Add stock and coconut milk, stir and bring to a boil.
4. Add red bell pepper, chicken and fish sauce, stir and simmer for 4 minutes more.
5. Add cilantro, stir, cook for 1 minute and take off heat.
6. Divide zucchini noodles into soup bowls, add soup on top and serve with lime wedges on the side.

Enjoy!

Nutrition: calories 287, fat 14, fiber 2, carbs 7, protein 25

Delicious Lunch Curry

Have you ever tried a keto curry? Then pay attention next!

Preparation time: 10 minutes

Cooking time: 1 hour

Servings: 4

Ingredients:

- 3 tomatoes, chopped
- 2 tablespoons olive oil
- 1 cup chicken stock
- 14 ounces canned coconut milk
- 1 tablespoon lime juice
- Salt and black pepper to the taste
- 2 pounds chicken thighs, boneless and skinless and cubed
- 2 garlic cloves, minced
- 1 cup white onion, chopped
- 3 red chilies, chopped
- 1 ounce peanuts, toasted
- 1 tablespoon water
- 1 tablespoon ginger, grated

- 2 teaspoons coriander, ground
- 1 teaspoon cinnamon, ground
- 1 teaspoon turmeric, ground
- 1 teaspoon cumin, ground
- ½ teaspoon black pepper
- 1 teaspoon fennel seeds, ground

Directions:

1. In your food processor, mix white onion with garlic, peanuts, red chilies, water, ginger, coriander, cinnamon, turmeric, cumin, fennel and black pepper, blend until you obtain a paste and leave aside for now.
2. Heat up a pan with the olive oil over medium high heat, add spice paste you've made, stir well and heat up for a few seconds.
3. Add chicken pieces, stir and cook for 2 minutes.
4. Add stock and tomatoes, stir, reduce heat to low and cook for 30 minutes.

5. Add coconut milk, stir and cook for 20 minutes more.

6. Add salt, pepper and lime juice, stir, divide into bowls and serve.

Enjoy!

Nutrition: calories 430, fat 22, fiber 4, carbs 7, protein 53

Lunch Spinach Rolls

These will be ready in no time!

Preparation time: 20 minutes

Cooking time: 15 minutes

Servings: 16

Ingredients:

- 6 tablespoons coconut flour
- ½ cup almond flour
- 2 and ½ cups mozzarella cheese, shredded
- 2 eggs
- A pinch of salt

For the filling:

- 4 ounces cream cheese
- 6 ounces spinach, torn
- A drizzle of avocado oil
- A pinch of salt
- ¼ cup parmesan, grated
- Mayonnaise for serving

Directions:

1. Heat up a pan with the oil over medium heat, add spinach and cook for 2 minutes.
2. Add parmesan, a pinch of salt and cream cheese, stir well, take off heat and leave aside for now.
3. Put mozzarella cheese in a heatproof bowl and microwave for 30 seconds.
4. Add eggs, salt, coconut and almond flour and stir everything.
5. Place dough on a lined cutting board, place a parchment paper on top and flatten dough with a rolling pin.
6. Divide dough into 16 rectangles, spread spinach mix on each and roll them into cigar shapes.
7. Place all rolls on a lined baking sheet, introduce in the oven at 350 degrees F and bake for 15 minutes.
8. Leave rolls to cool down for a few minutes before serving them with some mayo on top.

Enjoy!

Nutrition: calories 500, fat 65, fiber 4, carbs 14, protein 32

Delicious Steak Bowl

It's an easy and fulfilling keto lunch! Try it!

Preparation time: 15 minutes

Cooking time: 8 minutes

Servings: 4

Ingredients:

- 16 ounces skirt steak
- 4 ounces pepper jack cheese, shredded
- 1 cup sour cream
- Salt and black pepper to the taste
- 1 handful cilantro, chopped
- A splash of chipotle adobo sauce

For the guacamole:

- ¼ cup red onion, chopped
- 2 avocados, pitted and peeled
- Juice from 1 lime
- 1 tablespoon olive oil
- 6 cherry tomatoes, chopped
- 1 garlic clove, minced

- 1 tablespoon cilantro, chopped
- Salt and black pepper to the taste

Directions:

1. Put avocados in a bowl and mash with a fork.
2. Add tomatoes, red onion, garlic, salt and pepper and stir well.
3. Add olive oil, lime juice and 1 tablespoon cilantro, stir again very well and leave aside for now.
4. Heat up a pan over high heat, add steak, season with salt and pepper, cook for 4 minutes on each side, transfer to a cutting board, leave aside to cool down a bit and cut into thin strips.
5. Divide steak into 4 bowls, add cheese, sour cream and guacamole on top and serve with a splash of chipotle adobo sauce.

Enjoy!

Nutrition: calories 600, fat 50, fiber 6, carbs 5, protein 30

Meatballs And Pilaf

This is a Ketogenic lunch everyone can enjoy!

Preparation time: 10 minutes

Cooking time: 30 minutes

Servings: 4

Ingredients:

- 12 ounces cauliflower florets
- Salt and black pepper to the taste
- 1 egg
- 1 pound lamb, ground
- 1 teaspoon fennel seed
- 1 teaspoon paprika
- 1 teaspoon garlic powder
- 1 small yellow onion, chopped
- 2 garlic cloves, minced
- 2 tablespoons coconut oil
- 1 bunch mint, chopped
- 1 tablespoon lemon zest
- 4 ounces goat cheese, crumbled

Directions:

1. Put cauliflower florets in your food processor, add salt and pulse well.
2. Grease a pan with some of the coconut oil, heat up over medium heat, add cauliflower rice, cook for 8 minutes, season with salt and pepper to the taste, take off heat and keep warm.
3. In a bowl, mix lamb with salt, pepper, egg, paprika, garlic powder and fennel seed and stir very well.
4. Shape 12 meatballs and place them on a plate for now.
5. Heat up a pan with the coconut oil over medium heat, add onion, stir and cook for 6 minutes.
6. Add garlic, stir and cook for 1 minute.
7. Add meatballs, cook them well on all sides and take off heat.
8. Divide cauliflower rice between plates, add meatballs and onion mix on top, sprinkle mint, lemon zest and goat cheese at the end and serve.

Enjoy!

Nutrition: calories 470, fat 43, fiber 5, carbs 4, protein 26

Lightning Source UK Ltd.
Milton Keynes UK
UKHW021856220421
382471UK00003B/246